ESSENTIAL GUIDE TO NECROBIOSIS LIPOIDICA

Comprehensive Insights and Management Strategies for a Rare Dermatological Condition

DR. CASEY LOREN

DISCLAIMER

This book's content is only meant to be used for general informative purposes. Although the author has taken great care to ensure the content is accurate and thorough, no warranties or assurances on the information's accuracy, correctness, or reliability are provided. It is recommended that readers employ their own judgment and discretion when applying any material found in this book to their particular situation.

The information in this book is not intended to replace professional advice, nor is the author an expert in any of the subjects covered. It is recommended that readers consult with experienced professionals regarding any particular issues or concerns.

Any name that may be mentioned or referred in this book does not imply endorsement, recommendation, or relationship on the part of the author with any person, entity, good, website, or association. These references are made only for informational purposes and are not meant to be taken as recommendations or endorsements.

The information contained in this book may cause readers to suffer loss or damage, for which the author disclaims all obligation and accountability. The only people accountable for the decisions and actions taken by readers using the information presented are themselves.

Any names, characters, companies, locations, activities, occasions, and incidents referenced in this book are either made up or the result of the author's imagination. Any likeness to real people, living or dead, or to real things is entirely coincidental.

This book's content may change at any time, without prior notice, according to the author. The onus is on the reader to verify whether there have been any updates or revisions.

The reader accepts the conditions of this disclaimer by reading this book. Please do not

read this book or use its contents if you do not
agree to these terms.

CHAPTER 1

INTRODUCTION TO NECROBIOSIS LIPOIDICA

Overview of Necrobiosis Lipoidica

Necrobiosis Lipoidica (NL) is a rare, chronic skin disorder characterized by yellowish-brown, atrophic plaques, most commonly found on the shins. The condition is thought to be related to abnormal collagen and blood vessel changes in the skin. Although the exact cause is unknown, NL is frequently associated with diabetes mellitus, with up to 11-65% of patients also having diabetes. The plaques can be asymptomatic or painful and ulcerate, leading to complications and requiring medical intervention. Understanding NL involves recognizing its clinical presentation, potential complications, and the importance of interdisciplinary management in affected patients.

Historical Background

Necrobiosis Lipoidica was first described in 1929 by Urbach, a German dermatologist. Initially observed in patients with diabetes, the condition was later recognized in non-diabetic individuals as well. Historical descriptions have evolved with an improved understanding of its pathophysiology, aided by advancements in dermatological research and diagnostic techniques. The progression in the recognition and management of NL reflects broader trends in medical science, emphasizing the integration of clinical observation with laboratory research.

Epidemiology and Prevalence

NL affects an estimated 0.3% of the general population, with a higher prevalence among individuals with diabetes, particularly type 1 diabetes. It typically manifests in adults aged 20-60, with a higher incidence in females. Epidemiological studies suggest that about 11-65% of those with NL have diabetes, though NL can also occur in non-diabetic individuals. The exact prevalence may be underreported due to misdiagnosis or the asymptomatic nature of early lesions. Understanding the epidemiology is crucial for recognizing at-risk populations and implementing early interventions.

Importance of Awareness

Raising awareness about NL is vital for early diagnosis and management, particularly among healthcare providers and patients with diabetes. Awareness can lead to timely recognition, reducing the risk of complications such as ulceration and secondary infections. Educating patients about the condition can improve adherence to treatment plans and promote proactive skin care. Increased awareness also encourages research funding and support for those affected by NL, fostering better outcomes through enhanced medical and community support.

Differences Between Necrobiosis Lipoidica and Other Skin Conditions

NL can be mistaken for other dermatological conditions, such as granuloma annulare, diabetic dermopathy, and venous stasis dermatitis. Key differentiators include the appearance of lesions (yellowish-brown, atrophic plaques with telangiectasia), the typical location (shins), and the association with diabetes. Granuloma annulare usually presents as annular plaques without atrophy, while diabetic dermopathy manifests as smaller, pigmented patches. Accurate diagnosis involves clinical evaluation and sometimes biopsy to distinguish NL from these and other conditions.

Goals of This Guide

The primary goal of this guide is to provide comprehensive information about NL, enhancing understanding and management of the condition. We aim to:

1. Educate healthcare professionals and patients about NL's clinical features, diagnosis, and treatment.

2. Highlight the importance of early recognition and intervention to prevent complications.

3. Address common misconceptions and myths surrounding NL.

4. Share personal stories and case studies to illustrate the real-life impact of NL.

5. Encourage a multidisciplinary approach to managing NL, involving dermatologists, endocrinologists, and other specialists.

Personal Stories and Case Studies

Personal stories and case studies provide valuable insights into the lived experiences of those with NL. They highlight the challenges of diagnosis, treatment journeys, and the psychological and social impacts of the condition. For example, a case study might detail the experience of a patient with type 1 diabetes who developed NL and the subsequent management strategies employed to control the disease. These narratives offer practical lessons and inspire both patients and healthcare providers to pursue effective care strategies.

Common Myths and Misconceptions

Several myths and misconceptions surround NL, including:

1. **Myth:** NL only affects people with diabetes.

   Fact: While commonly associated with diabetes, NL can occur in non-diabetic individuals.

2. **Myth:** NL is always painful.

   Fact: NL can be asymptomatic or painful, depending on the stage and presence of ulceration.

3. **Myth:** There is no effective treatment for NL.

Fact: While challenging to treat, several therapies, including topical steroids, systemic treatments, and laser therapy, can manage symptoms and improve skin appearance.

The Role of Dermatology in Diagnosis

Dermatologists play a crucial role in diagnosing NL through clinical examination and, when necessary, skin biopsies. Their expertise helps differentiate NL from other dermatological conditions, ensuring appropriate management. Dermatologists also guide patients through treatment options, monitoring progress and adjusting therapies as needed. Collaboration with other specialists, such as endocrinologists, is often essential for comprehensive care, especially in patients with diabetes.

How This Book Is Organized

This guide is structured to provide a thorough understanding of NL, from basic information to advanced management strategies. The chapters include:

1. **Introduction:** An overview of NL and its significance.

2. **Clinical Features:** Detailed descriptions of NL's presentation and differential diagnoses.

3. **Diagnostic Approaches:** Tools and techniques for accurate diagnosis.

4. **Treatment Options:** Current and emerging therapies for NL.

5. **Patient Perspectives:** Personal stories and case studies.

6. **Myths and Misconceptions:** Addressing common misunderstandings about NL.

7. **Interdisciplinary Management:** The role of various healthcare providers in managing NL.

8. **Future Directions:** Research trends and potential advancements in NL treatment.

This organization ensures a logical flow of information, guiding readers from foundational knowledge to practical applications in managing Necrobiosis Lipoidica.

CHAPTER 2

UNDERSTANDING THE CAUSES

Understanding the Causes of Necrobiosis Lipoidica

Necrobiosis Lipoidica (NL) is a chronic skin condition characterized by the development of yellowish-brown patches, primarily on the shins. While the exact cause of NL remains unknown, various factors are believed to contribute to its development. This comprehensive guide explores the potential causes and contributing factors of NL.

Genetic Factors

Genetic predisposition plays a role in the development of NL, though the specific genetic markers have not been identified. Studies suggest that individuals with a family history of autoimmune diseases, including NL, may have a higher risk of developing the condition. Genetic research continues to explore the heritable aspects of NL to identify potential genetic links.

Immune System Involvement

NL is considered to be an immune-mediated condition. It is thought to involve an abnormal immune response that leads to inflammation and degeneration of collagen in the skin. This process results in the characteristic lesions of NL. Autoimmune disorders, where the immune system attacks the body's tissues, are often associated with NL, further supporting the role of immune system involvement.

Environmental Triggers

Environmental factors may act as triggers for the onset or exacerbation of NL. These can include:

- Trauma to the skin, such as cuts or abrasions

- Prolonged sun exposure

- Exposure to certain chemicals or allergens

While these factors do not cause NL directly, they can initiate or worsen the inflammatory response in predisposed individuals.

Hormonal Influences

Hormonal changes and imbalances may influence the development of NL. Observations indicate that NL can be more prevalent in females, suggesting a potential link to hormonal factors. However, the exact mechanisms by which hormones affect NL are not fully understood and require further investigation.

The Role of Diabetes

There is a well-documented association between NL and diabetes mellitus. Approximately one-third to one-half of individuals with NL have diabetes. The exact reason for this link is unclear, but it is believed that vascular changes and impaired glucose metabolism in diabetes contribute to the development of NL lesions. Good glycemic control is essential for managing NL in diabetic patients.

Lifestyle and Dietary Factors

Lifestyle and dietary habits can impact the progression of NL, especially in individuals with diabetes. Factors such as:

- Poor blood sugar control

- Obesity

- Lack of physical activity

Can exacerbate NL. Adopting a healthy lifestyle with a balanced diet and regular exercise can help manage symptoms and prevent complications.

Impact of Stress

Stress is known to affect the immune system and exacerbate many skin conditions, including NL. Chronic stress can lead to increased inflammation and may worsen NL symptoms. Stress management techniques, such as mindfulness, relaxation exercises, and counseling, can be beneficial for patients with NL.

Infections and Necrobiosis Lipoidica

Certain infections have been implicated in the development of NL. Bacterial, viral, and fungal infections can trigger an immune response that may lead to the formation of NL lesions. Identifying and treating underlying infections can be an important aspect of managing NL.

Coexisting Conditions

NL often coexists with other medical conditions, which can complicate its management. Conditions commonly associated with NL include:

- Autoimmune diseases (e.g., rheumatoid arthritis, lupus)

- Peripheral vascular disease

- Thyroid disorders

Understanding and addressing these coexisting conditions are crucial for comprehensive care.

Ongoing Research on Causes

Research into the causes of NL is ongoing. Current studies focus on:

- Identifying specific genetic markers associated with NL

- Understanding the immune mechanisms involved in NL

- Exploring the impact of metabolic factors, such as insulin resistance, on NL

- Investigating the role of environmental and lifestyle factors in triggering NL

Advancements in research may lead to better diagnostic tools, targeted therapies, and improved outcomes for individuals with NL.

Understanding the multifaceted causes of Necrobiosis Lipoidica is essential for developing effective management strategies. While genetic, immune, environmental, hormonal, and lifestyle factors all play a role, ongoing research continues to shed light on the complex interactions that contribute to this condition. By staying informed and adopting comprehensive care approaches, patients and healthcare providers can work together to manage and mitigate the impact of NL.

CHAPTER 3

SYMPTOMS AND DIAGNOSIS

Identifying Early Symptoms

Necrobiosis lipoidica (NL) is a rare, chronic skin condition often associated with diabetes mellitus. Early symptoms typically present as small, red, or brownish-yellow papules or plaques, most commonly appearing on the shins. These lesions are usually asymptomatic, meaning they do not cause pain or discomfort initially. Other early signs include:

- Shiny, atrophic skin over the lesions

- Telangiectasia (visible small blood vessels) on the surface

- Pruritus (itching), although less common in early stages

Progression of the Disease

As NL progresses, the lesions may expand and merge to form larger plaques with distinct, raised, and waxy borders. The center of these plaques may become depressed, taking on a yellowish hue. Over time, the skin within these plaques can become thin, ulcerated, and prone to infection. Key stages in disease progression include:

- Enlargement and coalescence of initial lesions

- Central yellowish atrophy with red-brown borders

- Potential ulceration, which can lead to secondary infections

Physical Examination Techniques

During a physical examination, a dermatologist will look for characteristic features of NL. Important aspects include:

- Inspecting the lower legs, especially the shins

- Assessing the size, color, and texture of the lesions

- Checking for signs of ulceration or secondary infection

- Noting any telangiectasia or atrophic changes

A thorough physical examination can help differentiate NL from other dermatological conditions with similar presentations.

Skin Biopsy Procedure

A skin biopsy is often necessary to confirm the diagnosis of NL. The procedure involves:

1. Local anesthesia is applied to the lesion site.

2. A small sample of the affected skin is removed using a punch or excisional biopsy technique.

3. The tissue sample is sent to a laboratory for histopathological examination.

Histological findings characteristic of NL include:

- Granulomatous inflammation

- Degeneration of collagen (necrobiosis)

- Thickened blood vessel walls

Differential Diagnosis

Differential diagnosis is crucial to distinguish NL from other conditions with similar symptoms. Conditions to consider include:

- Diabetic dermopathy

- Granuloma annulare

- Sarcoidosis

- Erythema nodosum

- Lichen planus

- Xanthomas

Each of these conditions has distinct histological and clinical features that can help in differentiation.

Imaging Studies

While not always necessary, imaging studies can be helpful in certain cases:

- **Doppler Ultrasound**: To assess blood flow and detect any vascular abnormalities in the affected area.

- **MRI**: In rare cases, MRI can help evaluate deeper tissue involvement and rule out other conditions.

Laboratory Tests

Laboratory tests are often conducted to rule out underlying systemic conditions and support the diagnosis of NL:

- **Blood glucose levels**: Given the strong association with diabetes, testing for hyperglycemia is essential.

- **HbA1c**: This test measures long-term blood glucose control.

- **Lipid profile**: To check for dyslipidemia, which may be associated with NL.

- **Inflammatory markers**: Such as ESR and CRP, although these are typically normal in NL.

The Role of Medical History

A comprehensive medical history is vital for diagnosing NL. Key aspects to cover include:

- History of diabetes or glucose intolerance

- Duration and control of diabetes

- Family history of NL or other skin conditions

- History of trauma or infection in the affected area

- Review of any other systemic symptoms or conditions

Common Diagnostic Challenges

Diagnosing NL can be challenging due to its rarity and the overlap with other dermatological conditions. Common challenges include:

- Atypical presentations, such as lesions on areas other than the shins

- Misdiagnosis as diabetic dermopathy, especially in diabetic patients

- Difficulty in obtaining a sufficient biopsy sample from atrophic or ulcerated lesions

Patient Experiences with Diagnosis

Patients often report a prolonged diagnostic journey, marked by visits to multiple specialists and undergoing various tests before receiving a definitive diagnosis. Common experiences include:

- Initial misdiagnoses and ineffective treatments

- Emotional distress due to the chronic nature and cosmetic impact of the disease

- Relief upon finally receiving an accurate diagnosis, which can lead to more targeted and effective management strategies

Overall, a multidisciplinary approach involving dermatologists, endocrinologists, and other specialists is often required to accurately diagnose and manage NL, ensuring comprehensive care for affected patients.

CHAPTER 4

TREATMENT OPTIONS

Essential Guide to Necrobiosis Lipoidica: Treatment Options

Necrobiosis lipoidica (NL) is a rare, chronic skin condition characterized by the development of yellow, waxy plaques, usually on the lower legs. Effective management requires a comprehensive understanding of various treatment options. Here, we delve into each available treatment method to provide a thorough understanding.

Topical Treatments

1. Corticosteroids: Topical corticosteroids are commonly used to reduce inflammation and slow the progression of lesions. These can be applied directly to the affected areas. Potent corticosteroids may be necessary for more severe cases, but long-term use can lead to skin thinning.

2. Calcineurin Inhibitors: Topical tacrolimus or pimecrolimus can be alternatives to corticosteroids, especially for facial or sensitive areas. These agents modulate the immune response and can be effective in reducing inflammation with a lower risk of skin atrophy.

3. Moisturizers: Emollients and moisturizers help maintain skin hydration and integrity, which is crucial for preventing further damage and improving overall skin health.

Systemic Medications

1. Oral Corticosteroids: For severe cases, systemic corticosteroids like prednisone may be prescribed. These help to rapidly reduce inflammation but are associated with significant side effects such as weight gain, osteoporosis, and increased infection risk.

2. Immunosuppressants: Drugs such as methotrexate or azathioprine are used to manage NL by suppressing the immune system. These are typically reserved for cases unresponsive to other treatments due to their potential for serious side effects.

3. Antimalarials: Hydroxychloroquine has shown some efficacy in treating NL due to its anti-inflammatory and immunomodulatory properties.

4. Pentoxifylline: This medication improves blood flow and has anti-inflammatory effects, making it useful in managing NL, particularly when there is significant vascular involvement.

Steroid Injections

Intralesional Steroids: Injecting corticosteroids directly into the lesions can help reduce inflammation and flatten plaques. This method can be particularly effective for localized areas, though repeated treatments may be necessary.

Laser Therapy

1. Pulsed Dye Laser (PDL): This laser targets blood vessels in the skin, reducing redness and improving the appearance of lesions. It is particularly useful for the erythematous (red) phase of NL.

2. Ablative and Non-ablative Lasers: These lasers can help resurface the skin and improve texture. Ablative lasers remove layers of skin, while non-ablative lasers stimulate collagen production without significant surface damage.

Phototherapy

1. UVA1 Therapy: This type of phototherapy uses long-wave ultraviolet A light, which penetrates deeper into the skin and can help reduce inflammation and improve lesions.

2. PUVA Therapy: Combines psoralen (a photosensitizing agent) with UVA light. It is effective for various skin conditions, including NL, but carries a risk of skin aging and cancer with long-term use.

Surgical Interventions

1. Excision and Grafting: In cases of extensive or refractory NL, surgical removal of lesions followed by skin grafting may be considered. This is typically a last resort due to the risk of complications such as infection or poor wound healing.

2. Debridement: Removal of necrotic or ulcerated tissue can promote healing and reduce the risk of secondary infections.

Alternative and Complementary Therapies

1. Herbal Remedies: Some herbal treatments, such as aloe vera or turmeric, have anti-inflammatory properties. However, their efficacy in NL is not well-documented, and they should be used with caution.

2. Acupuncture: This traditional Chinese medicine technique may help manage symptoms by improving blood flow and reducing pain, though evidence of its effectiveness in NL is limited.

3. Dietary Supplements: Omega-3 fatty acids, vitamin E, and antioxidants might help reduce inflammation and improve skin health, though their specific benefits for NL need further research.

Managing Side Effects

1. Skin Atrophy: Long-term corticosteroid use can lead to skin thinning. Using the lowest effective dose and limiting duration can mitigate this risk.

2. Systemic Effects: Oral and systemic treatments can cause a range of side effects, from gastrointestinal issues to immunosuppression. Regular monitoring and preventive measures, such as bone density scans for osteoporosis, are crucial.

3. Infection Risk: Immunosuppressive therapies increase infection risk. Patients should be advised on infection prevention and monitored for signs of infection.

Treatment for Coexisting Conditions

1. Diabetes Management: As NL is often associated with diabetes, optimizing blood glucose control is essential. This can help reduce the severity of NL and improve overall outcomes.

2. Vascular Health: Addressing any underlying vascular issues, such as peripheral artery disease, can improve skin perfusion and support healing.

3. Autoimmune Conditions: Patients with other autoimmune disorders may require coordinated care to manage overlapping symptoms and treatments effectively.

Ongoing Research in Treatments

1. Biological Therapies: Research is ongoing into the use of biologics, which target specific pathways in the immune system. These could offer new avenues for treating NL with potentially fewer side effects than traditional immunosuppressants.

2. Gene Therapy: Investigations into the genetic basis of NL may lead to gene-targeted treatments, offering personalized and effective options.

3. Novel Topicals: Development of new topical agents that target specific inflammatory pathways or promote skin regeneration is an active area of research.

4. Clinical Trials: Participation in clinical trials can provide access to cutting-edge treatments and contribute to the broader understanding of NL management.

In conclusion, managing Necrobiosis Lipoidica requires a multifaceted approach tailored to the individual patient. A combination of topical treatments, systemic medications, and adjunctive therapies, alongside careful management of side effects and coexisting conditions, offers the best chance for successful outcomes. Ongoing research continues to expand the therapeutic options available, providing hope for more effective and targeted treatments in the future.

CHAPTER 5

LIVING WITH NECROBIOSIS LIPOIDICA

Necrobiosis Lipoidica (NL) is a rare, chronic skin condition often associated with diabetes, characterized by red-brown, yellow, or waxy patches on the skin, typically on the shins. Managing NL requires a comprehensive approach to skincare, symptom management, and lifestyle adjustments. This guide provides an extensive overview of essential aspects to consider for those living with NL.

Daily Skincare Routines

Cleansing and Moisturizing

- **Gentle Cleansing:** Use mild, fragrance-free cleansers to avoid irritation. Harsh soaps can strip natural oils and exacerbate dryness.

- **Moisturizing:** Apply a thick, hypoallergenic moisturizer immediately after bathing to lock in moisture. Consider products with ceramides or hyaluronic acid for added hydration.

Sun Protection

- **Sunscreen:** Use broad-spectrum sunscreen with at least SPF 30 daily to protect affected areas from UV damage, which can worsen lesions.

- **Protective Clothing:** Wear long pants and socks to shield your skin from the sun.

Specialized Care

- **Topical Treatments:** Your dermatologist may prescribe corticosteroids or other topical treatments to reduce inflammation and slow disease progression.

- **Monitoring Changes:** Regularly check your skin for new lesions or changes in existing ones. Early detection of changes can lead to prompt medical intervention.

Managing Symptoms at Home

Symptom Alleviation

- **Pain Management:** Over-the-counter pain relievers like acetaminophen or ibuprofen can help manage discomfort.

- **Itch Relief:** Antihistamines or topical anti-itch creams can alleviate itching.

Wound Care

- **Infection Prevention:** Keep lesions clean and covered with sterile bandages if they are open or weeping. Use antibiotic ointments as directed by your healthcare provider.

- **Hydration:** Maintain good skin hydration to promote healing and prevent cracking or bleeding.

Coping with Physical Changes

Aesthetic Concerns

- **Camouflage Techniques:** Consider using medical-grade makeup to cover lesions if their appearance causes distress. Color-correcting creams can neutralize red or yellow tones.

- **Clothing Choices:** Opt for clothing that covers affected areas comfortably, avoiding tight or abrasive fabrics that might irritate the skin.

Physical Discomfort

- **Footwear:** Wear supportive, comfortable shoes that don't rub against lesions on your shins or feet.

Psychological Impact and Mental Health

Emotional Support

- **Counseling:** Consider professional counseling or therapy to address feelings of self-consciousness, anxiety, or depression.

- **Mindfulness Practices:** Techniques such as meditation, deep-breathing exercises, or yoga can help manage stress and improve overall mental well-being.

Social Interaction

- **Open Communication:** Talk openly with friends and family about your condition to foster understanding and support.

- **Peer Support:** Engage with others who have NL through support groups or online communities to share experiences and coping strategies.

Support Systems and Communities

Family and Friends

- **Education:** Educate your loved ones about NL so they can provide informed support.

- **Involvement:** Encourage family and friends to accompany you to medical appointments or participate in your care routines.

Professional Support

- **Healthcare Team:** Build a multidisciplinary team including dermatologists, endocrinologists, and mental health professionals.

- **Support Groups:** Join local or online support groups for people with NL to connect with others facing similar challenges.

Lifestyle Modifications

Diabetes Management

- **Blood Sugar Control:** If you have diabetes, maintaining stable blood sugar levels is crucial as high levels can exacerbate NL.

- **Regular Monitoring:** Keep track of your glucose levels and follow your diabetes management plan diligently.

Healthy Habits

- **No Smoking:** Avoid smoking as it can worsen skin conditions and impede healing.

- **Moderate Alcohol:** Limit alcohol consumption, as excessive drinking can negatively impact overall health and skin integrity.

Importance of Regular Medical Check-ups

Routine Examinations

- **Dermatological Visits:** Regularly see your dermatologist to monitor NL progression and adjust treatments as needed.

- **Comprehensive Check-ups:** Schedule regular check-ups with your primary care physician to manage underlying conditions, such as diabetes or vascular issues.

Early Intervention

- **Prompt Treatment:** Address new symptoms or changes in lesions promptly with your healthcare provider to prevent complications.

Nutritional Considerations

Balanced Diet

- **Anti-Inflammatory Foods:** Incorporate foods rich in antioxidants, omega-3 fatty acids, and vitamins C and E to help reduce inflammation and support skin health.

- **Hydration:** Drink plenty of water to keep your skin hydrated from the inside out.

Dietary Adjustments

- **Low-Glycemic Foods:** If you have diabetes, focus on low-glycemic foods to help maintain stable blood sugar levels.

- **Nutritional Supplements:** Discuss with your healthcare provider whether supplements like vitamin D or zinc might benefit your condition.

Exercise and Physical Activity

Regular Exercise

- **Low-Impact Activities:** Engage in low-impact exercises such as walking, swimming, or cycling to improve circulation without stressing your skin.

- **Strength and Flexibility:** Incorporate strength training and flexibility exercises to support overall health and well-being.

Precautions

- **Protective Gear:** Wear appropriate clothing and protective gear to avoid skin injury during physical activity.

- **Post-Exercise Care:** Cleanse and moisturize your skin after exercising to remove sweat and prevent irritation.

Long-term Outlook

Disease Progression

- **Monitoring:** Regular follow-ups with your healthcare team can help manage NL effectively and monitor for potential complications.

- **Research and Treatments:** Stay informed about new research and emerging treatments that may offer additional options for managing NL.

Quality of Life

- **Adaptation:** Focus on adapting your lifestyle to manage symptoms and maintain a good quality of life.

- **Proactive Management:** Taking a proactive approach to healthcare, skincare, and mental health can significantly improve long-term outcomes.

Living with Necrobiosis Lipoidica can be challenging, but with comprehensive care and support, individuals can manage their symptoms and maintain a fulfilling life. Regular medical care, proper skin care, emotional support, and lifestyle adjustments are key components in managing this condition effectively.

CHAPTER 6

THE ROLE OF HEALTHCARE PROVIDERS

Dermatologists and Their Role

Dermatologists are key players in diagnosing and managing Necrobiosis Lipoidica (NL), a chronic skin condition often associated with diabetes. Their expertise in skin disorders enables them to identify NL through clinical examination and, if necessary, skin biopsies. Dermatologists manage the condition by prescribing topical or systemic treatments, including corticosteroids, immunomodulators, or biologics. They also monitor for potential complications like ulcerations or secondary infections and collaborate with other specialists to ensure comprehensive care.

Endocrinologists and Diabetes Management

Endocrinologists specialize in hormone-related diseases, including diabetes, which is frequently linked to NL. Their role involves managing blood glucose levels to minimize the risk of complications that could exacerbate NL. They may adjust insulin therapy or other diabetic medications, provide dietary and lifestyle recommendations, and monitor for complications such as neuropathy or retinopathy. Effective diabetes management by endocrinologists is crucial in controlling NL and improving patient outcomes.

Primary Care Physicians

Primary care physicians (PCPs) often serve as the first point of contact for patients with NL. They play a crucial role in early detection and referral to specialists like dermatologists and endocrinologists. PCPs manage overall health, monitor chronic conditions, and provide patient education on lifestyle modifications to control diabetes. They coordinate care among specialists, ensuring a holistic approach to the patient's health.

Role of Nurses and Medical Staff

Nurses and medical staff are integral to the day-to-day management of NL and diabetes. They provide patient education on wound care, medication administration, and lifestyle changes. Nurses also monitor patient progress, manage routine follow-ups, and offer emotional support. Their role extends to educating patients about the importance of skincare and diabetes management, helping to prevent complications, and improving quality of life.

Importance of a Multidisciplinary Approach

NL requires a multidisciplinary approach due to its complex nature and association with systemic conditions like diabetes. This approach involves collaboration among dermatologists, endocrinologists, PCPs, nurses, podiatrists, and sometimes vascular surgeons. Each specialist addresses different aspects of the disease, from skin management to systemic control of diabetes and wound care. A multidisciplinary team ensures comprehensive care, addressing all facets of the patient's health.

Communication with Healthcare Providers

Effective communication between patients and healthcare providers is crucial in managing NL. Patients should be encouraged to ask questions, express concerns, and share their experiences. Clear communication helps in understanding the treatment plan, adherence to medications, and lifestyle adjustments. Providers should use layman's terms, offer written materials, and employ visual aids when necessary to enhance understanding.

Patient Advocacy

Patient advocacy involves empowering patients to take an active role in their healthcare. Advocates educate patients about their condition, treatment options, and rights within the healthcare system. They assist in navigating insurance issues and accessing necessary services. Advocacy groups can also provide support networks, resources, and information, helping patients manage NL more effectively.

Finding the Right Specialist

Finding the right specialist is essential for effective management of NL. Patients should seek referrals from their PCP or use reputable medical directories. It's important to consider specialists' experience with NL and diabetes. Patient reviews and recommendations from support groups can also be valuable. Ensuring the chosen specialist has a collaborative approach and communicates well is crucial for ongoing care.

Preparing for Medical Appointments

Preparation for medical appointments enhances the effectiveness of consultations. Patients should keep a detailed record of their symptoms, treatment history, and any changes in their condition. Bringing a list of questions, current medications, and relevant medical records is also beneficial. Being prepared helps patients make the most of their appointment time and ensures all concerns are addressed.

Navigating the Healthcare System

Navigating the healthcare system can be challenging for patients with NL. Understanding insurance coverage, referral processes, and accessing specialist care are critical steps. Patients should familiarize themselves with their insurance benefits and seek assistance from healthcare providers or patient advocates when needed. Keeping track of appointments, test results, and treatment plans is also essential for effective disease management. Using digital health tools and patient portals can simplify these tasks and enhance communication with healthcare providers.

In summary, managing Necrobiosis Lipoidica requires a comprehensive, coordinated approach involving various healthcare providers. Each plays a distinct role, from initial diagnosis and treatment to ongoing management and patient support, ensuring the best possible outcomes for patients.

CHAPTER 7

NECROBIOSIS LIPOIDICA AND DIABETES

Understanding the Link Between Diabetes and Necrobiosis Lipoidica

Necrobiosis Lipoidica (NL) is a chronic skin condition that manifests as yellow, brown, or red patches on the skin, typically on the shins. The exact cause of NL is not well understood, but it is closely associated with diabetes, particularly type 1 diabetes. Up to 0.3% of diabetics may develop NL. The condition is believed to be linked to changes in blood vessels due to high blood sugar levels, leading to thickening of the blood vessel walls and subsequent decreased blood supply to the skin. This results in inflammation and degradation of collagen, causing the characteristic lesions of NL.

Diabetes Management Strategies

Effective management of diabetes is crucial in preventing and mitigating NL. Key strategies include:

- **Blood Glucose Monitoring**: Regular monitoring of blood sugar levels helps in maintaining them within a target range.

- **Medication Adherence**: Ensuring consistent use of insulin or other prescribed diabetes medications.

- **Diet and Nutrition**: Following a balanced diet rich in fiber, low in refined sugars, and with controlled carbohydrate intake.

- **Exercise**: Engaging in regular physical activity to improve insulin sensitivity and overall health.

- **Regular Medical Check-ups**: Routine visits to healthcare providers for comprehensive diabetes management and early detection of complications.

Impact of Blood Sugar Levels on Skin Health

Chronic high blood sugar levels can damage small blood vessels, impairing blood circulation to the skin and leading to poor wound healing, dryness, and susceptibility to infections. In the case of NL, poor glycemic control exacerbates the condition, making lesions more pronounced and difficult to heal. Maintaining optimal blood sugar levels is essential for preserving skin integrity and preventing the progression of skin conditions associated with diabetes.

Monitoring for Complications

Patients with diabetes should be vigilant about skin changes and other potential complications. Regular self-examinations and professional skin evaluations are recommended. Signs to watch for include:

- Persistent lesions or ulcers that do not heal

- Changes in the color or size of NL patches

- Signs of infection such as increased redness, warmth, or discharge

Early intervention can prevent severe complications and promote better outcomes.

Coordinating Care Between Dermatologists and Endocrinologists

Effective management of NL in diabetic patients requires a multidisciplinary approach. Dermatologists and endocrinologists must collaborate closely to:

- Develop comprehensive treatment plans addressing both skin and systemic health.

- Adjust diabetes management strategies to optimize blood glucose control.

- Monitor for potential side effects of treatments and adjust as necessary.

- Provide patient education on maintaining skin health and preventing complications.

Case Studies of Diabetes-Related Necrobiosis Lipoidica

Case studies offer valuable insights into the presentation and management of NL in diabetic patients. They typically include:

- Patient history and diabetes management background

- Clinical presentation of NL lesions

- Diagnostic approaches such as biopsy and imaging

- Treatment interventions and outcomes

These studies highlight the importance of individualized care and the potential benefits of innovative therapies.

Preventative Measures for Diabetic Patients

Preventative strategies can reduce the risk of developing NL or mitigate its severity. These include:

- Strict blood glucose control through lifestyle and medication management

- Regular skin care routines to maintain hydration and prevent dryness

- Protective measures to avoid skin trauma, especially on the shins

- Timely treatment of skin infections or injuries to prevent complications

Patient Education on Diabetes and Skin Health

Educating patients about the connection between diabetes and skin health is crucial. Key educational points include:

- Importance of blood sugar control in preventing skin conditions

- Recognizing early signs of NL and other diabetes-related skin issues

- Proper skin care practices, including moisturizing and sun protection

- When to seek medical advice for skin changes

Recent Advances in Diabetes Research

Recent research has focused on understanding the pathophysiology of diabetes and its complications, including skin conditions like NL. Advances include:

- Development of novel medications and therapies for better glycemic control

- Insights into the genetic and molecular mechanisms linking diabetes to skin disorders

- Innovations in wound healing technologies and skin regeneration

- Improved diagnostic tools for early detection of diabetes-related complications

Personal Stories from Diabetic Patients

Personal narratives from diabetic patients with NL provide a human perspective on managing the condition. These stories often cover:

- The initial diagnosis and emotional impact

- Challenges faced in managing both diabetes and NL

- Successful strategies and treatments

- Support systems and resources that have been helpful

These accounts can inspire and educate others facing similar challenges, fostering a sense of community and shared experience.

By understanding the intricate relationship between diabetes and Necrobiosis Lipoidica, patients and healthcare providers can work together to achieve better health outcomes and improve quality of life.

CHAPTER 8
RESEARCH AND FUTURE DIRECTIONS

Current Research Trends

Current research on Necrobiosis Lipoidica (NL) focuses on understanding the pathophysiology, epidemiology, and optimal management strategies for this chronic skin condition. Researchers are exploring the following areas:

1. **Pathogenesis**: Investigations into the underlying mechanisms, including the role of immune system dysfunction, microangiopathy, and collagen degeneration.

2. **Epidemiology**: Studies aimed at determining the prevalence of NL in various populations and identifying risk factors associated with the condition, such as diabetes.

3. **Management**: Evaluating the effectiveness of existing treatments and identifying new therapeutic approaches.

4. **Quality of Life**: Assessing the impact of NL on patients' psychological and physical well-being.

Breakthroughs in Understanding Necrobiosis Lipoidica

Recent breakthroughs have shed light on several critical aspects of NL:

1. **Molecular Mechanisms**: Discovery of specific cytokines and growth factors involved in the inflammatory process.

2. **Genetic Predisposition**: Identification of genetic markers that may predispose individuals to NL, particularly in diabetic patients.

3. **Immunological Insights**: Understanding the role of immune cells, such as T-cells and macrophages, in the progression of NL lesions.

4. **Improved Imaging**: Advances in imaging techniques, such as dermoscopy and high-frequency ultrasound, have enhanced the visualization of NL lesions and their vascular components.

Emerging Treatments and Therapies

The landscape of NL treatment is evolving with several promising therapies on the horizon:

1. **Biologics**: Targeted biologic therapies, such as TNF inhibitors and IL-17 inhibitors, have shown potential in reducing inflammation and halting disease progression.

2. **Laser Therapy**: Use of vascular lasers, like the pulsed dye laser (PDL), to reduce erythema and improve lesion appearance.

3. **Topical Treatments**: Development of new topical agents, including immunomodulators and growth factor formulations.

4. **Systemic Therapies**: Exploration of systemic immunosuppressants and anti-inflammatory drugs for severe or refractory cases.

Genetic Studies and Findings

Genetic research has unveiled important insights into the hereditary aspects of NL:

1. **Genome-Wide Association Studies (GWAS)**: Identifying genetic variants linked to increased susceptibility to NL.

2. **Familial Studies**: Investigating the occurrence of NL in families to understand inheritance patterns and genetic predisposition.

3. **Gene Expression Profiling**: Analyzing gene expression in NL lesions to pinpoint key genetic drivers of the disease.

Innovations in Diagnostic Techniques

Innovative diagnostic methods are enhancing the accuracy and early detection of NL:

1. **Advanced Imaging**: Techniques such as confocal microscopy and optical coherence tomography (OCT) provide detailed imaging of skin layers and blood vessels.

2. **Biomarker Identification**: Research into serum and tissue biomarkers that can aid in the diagnosis and monitoring of NL.

3. **Non-Invasive Methods**: Development of non-invasive diagnostic tools to reduce the need for biopsies and improve patient comfort.

The Role of Clinical Trials

Clinical trials are pivotal in advancing NL research and treatment:

1. **Phase I-III Trials**: Evaluating the safety, efficacy, and optimal dosing of new treatments.

2. **Observational Studies**: Collecting data on the natural history and progression of NL to inform clinical practice.

3. **Patient Registries**: Establishing databases to track patient outcomes and identify patterns in treatment responses.

Contributions from Patient Advocacy Groups

Patient advocacy groups play a crucial role in NL research and awareness:

1. **Education and Awareness**: Raising public awareness about NL and providing educational resources for patients and healthcare providers.

2. **Funding Research**: Supporting research initiatives through fundraising and grant programs.

3. **Patient Support**: Offering support groups, counseling, and resources to help patients manage their condition and improve their quality of life.

4. **Policy Advocacy**: Advocating for policies that support NL research and ensure access to care for affected individuals.

Potential Future Cures

Research is ongoing to find a potential cure for NL:

1. **Stem Cell Therapy**: Investigating the use of stem cells to regenerate damaged skin and reduce inflammation.

2. **Gene Therapy**: Exploring the possibility of correcting genetic defects associated with NL.

3. **Novel Drug Development**: Developing new drugs that specifically target the molecular pathways involved in NL.

Ethical Considerations in Research

Ethical considerations are paramount in NL research:

1. **Informed Consent**: Ensuring patients are fully informed about the risks and benefits of participating in research.

2. **Privacy and Confidentiality**: Protecting the privacy of patient data and maintaining confidentiality.

3. **Equitable Access**: Ensuring all patients have equal access to participate in research studies and benefit from new treatments.

How to Get Involved in Research

Patients and healthcare providers can contribute to NL research in several ways:

1. **Clinical Trial Participation**: Patients can enroll in clinical trials to help test new treatments.

2. **Research Volunteering**: Volunteering for observational studies or patient registries.

3. **Advocacy and Fundraising**: Joining patient advocacy groups to support research efforts and raise funds.

4. **Professional Collaboration**: Healthcare providers can collaborate with research

institutions to recruit patients and share clinical data.

By staying informed and actively participating in research efforts, individuals and healthcare professionals can contribute to the advancement of knowledge and treatment options for Necrobiosis Lipoidica, ultimately improving outcomes for those affected by this condition.

CHAPTER 9

PERSONAL STORIES AND TESTIMONIALS

First-Hand Accounts from Patients:

1. **Understanding the Condition**: Patients often share their experiences of discovering Necrobiosis Lipoidica (NL) and how they navigated the initial confusion and concern.

2. **Symptom Challenges**: Detailed accounts about the physical symptoms they faced, including skin discoloration, lesions, and potential pain or itching.

3. **Emotional Impact**: Insights into the emotional toll NL can take, from frustration with misdiagnoses to anxiety about the condition's progression.

4. **Treatment Journey**: Personal narratives on trying different treatments, from topical creams

to more advanced therapies like steroid injections or immunosuppressive drugs.

5. **Management of Flare-Ups**: How patients manage and cope during flare-ups, including lifestyle adjustments and emotional support.

Stories of Diagnosis and Treatment Journeys:

1. **Early Symptoms and Concerns**: Patients recounting their initial symptoms and the process of seeking medical help.

2. **Medical Consultations**: Experiences with various healthcare professionals, from dermatologists to endocrinologists, and their roles in diagnosis and treatment planning.

3. **Treatment Successes and Setbacks**: Success stories about treatments that worked well, as well as challenges and setbacks faced along the way.

4. **Importance of Follow-Ups**: Emphasizing the significance of regular check-ups and

monitoring for disease progression or treatment adjustments.

Coping Strategies and Resilience:

1. **Emotional Coping**: Strategies for managing the emotional impact of living with NL, such as seeking support groups or therapy.

2. **Self-Care Practices**: Insights into self-care routines that help patients maintain their physical and mental well-being.

3. **Positive Mindset**: Stories highlighting the importance of maintaining a positive outlook and resilience despite the challenges NL presents.

Impact on Family and Friends:

1. **Family Dynamics**: How NL affects family relationships, including communication, support, and shared decision-making.

2. **Caregiver Perspectives**: Testimonials from caregivers about their experiences supporting a

loved one with NL and managing caregiving responsibilities.

3. **Educating Loved Ones**: Strategies for educating family and friends about NL to foster understanding and support.

Inspirational Recovery Stories:

1. **Overcoming Challenges**: Stories of individuals who have overcome significant obstacles related to NL and regained a sense of normalcy in their lives.

2. **Empowering Narratives**: How some patients turned their NL journey into a source of empowerment, advocacy, or creativity.

Lessons Learned from Personal Experiences:

1. **Medical Advocacy**: Insights into advocating for oneself within the healthcare system, including seeking second opinions and researching treatment options.

2. **Self-Discovery**: Personal growth and lessons learned about resilience, patience, and self-compassion through the NL journey.

Advice for Newly Diagnosed Patients:

1. **Seeking Information**: Encouragement to educate oneself about NL, its symptoms, treatments, and prognosis.

2. **Building Support Networks**: Advice on reaching out to healthcare professionals, support groups, and loved ones for guidance and support.

3. **Managing Expectations**: Setting realistic expectations about treatment outcomes and the unpredictable nature of NL.

Contributions from Caregivers:

1. **Caregiver Role**: Insights into the responsibilities and challenges of caregiving for someone with NL.

2. **Self-Care for Caregivers**: Advice for caregivers on prioritizing their well-being while supporting their loved ones.

Diverse Perspectives on Living with Necrobiosis Lipoidica:

1. **Age and Gender Variations**: How age and gender can impact the experience of living with NL, including differences in symptoms, treatments, and emotional responses.

2. **Cultural Influences**: Perspectives on how cultural beliefs and practices influence perceptions and management of NL.

3. **Work and Lifestyle Adjustments**: Stories about adapting work routines, hobbies, and social activities to accommodate NL symptoms and treatments.

Celebrating Triumphs and Overcoming Challenges:

1. **Milestones and Achievements**: Celebrating milestones in treatment progress, symptom management, and personal achievements despite NL challenges.

2. **Supportive Communities**: Recognition of the importance of support networks, advocacy groups, and online communities in celebrating successes and overcoming obstacles related to NL.

By incorporating these diverse personal stories and testimonials, the "ESSENTIAL GUIDE TO NECROBIOSIS LIPOIDICA" can provide a holistic and empathetic understanding of the condition, its impact, and strategies for coping and thriving despite its challenges.

CHAPTER 10
CONCLUSION AND FINAL THOUGHTS

Summary of Key Points

Necrobiosis lipoidica (NL) is a chronic skin condition characterized by red-brown, yellowish patches that typically appear on the lower legs. These lesions can ulcerate, causing pain and discomfort. The exact cause of NL is unknown, but it is often associated with diabetes. Diagnosis is primarily clinical but can be confirmed through a skin biopsy. Treatment options vary and include topical steroids, systemic treatments, and newer therapies such as biologics. Effective management requires a multidisciplinary approach, involving dermatologists, endocrinologists, and primary care providers.

Reflecting on the Journey with Necrobiosis Lipoidica

Living with NL can be challenging, both physically and emotionally. Patients often experience a range of feelings from frustration to hope as they navigate treatment options and lifestyle adjustments. The journey involves not only managing symptoms but also addressing the psychological impact of a visible skin condition. Understanding the progression of the disease, the effectiveness of various treatments, and coping strategies can significantly enhance the quality of life for those affected.

The Importance of Continued Awareness and Education

Raising awareness about NL is crucial. Many healthcare providers and the public remain unfamiliar with this condition, leading to misdiagnosis or delayed treatment. Education initiatives for medical professionals can improve early diagnosis and management, while public awareness campaigns can reduce stigma and support those living with NL. Educating patients empowers them to advocate for their care and make informed decisions about their treatment options.

Final Advice for Patients and Caregivers

For patients and caregivers, staying informed about NL is key. Keep up with the latest research, engage with support groups, and maintain open communication with healthcare providers. Self-care practices, such as proper skin care, balanced nutrition, and stress management, are vital. Caregivers should provide emotional support and encourage adherence to treatment plans, helping patients navigate the complexities of living with NL.

Emphasizing the Role of Research and Advocacy

Research is essential to advancing our understanding of NL and developing more effective treatments. Advocacy efforts can drive funding for research, influence healthcare policies, and ensure that the needs of patients with NL are addressed. Supporting organizations that focus on dermatological research and patient advocacy can make a significant impact.

How to Stay Updated with New Developments

Staying informed about new developments in NL can be achieved through several channels. Regularly review scientific journals, attend dermatology conferences, and join professional organizations dedicated to skin conditions. Online platforms, such as medical websites and social media groups, also provide updates and connect you with the broader community of patients and researchers.

Encouragement for the Future

While living with NL can be difficult, advances in medical research offer hope for better treatments and potential cures. Patients should remain optimistic and proactive in their care. Each discovery brings us closer to improved management and quality of life. Stay connected with support networks, and remember that progress in medicine often comes from the collective efforts of the community.

Gratitude for Contributors and Supporters

We extend our heartfelt gratitude to the researchers, healthcare providers, patient advocates, and everyone who has contributed to advancing our understanding of NL. Their dedication and hard work make a tangible difference in the lives of those affected by this condition. The support from families, friends, and caregivers also plays a crucial role in the well-being of patients.

Final Reflections from the Author

Writing this guide has been a journey of discovery and empathy. Understanding the complexities of NL and the resilience of those living with it has been enlightening. I hope that this guide serves as a valuable resource, providing clarity, support, and hope to patients, caregivers, and healthcare providers alike. Together, we can make strides towards better management and, ultimately, a cure for NL.

Resources for Further Support (excluding books)

- **American Academy of Dermatology (AAD):** Offers comprehensive information on NL and other skin conditions, including guidelines for treatment and patient education resources.

- **National Organization for Rare Disorders (NORD):** Provides resources and support for patients with rare conditions, including NL.

- **DermNet NZ:** A website dedicated to dermatological information, offering detailed descriptions, images, and treatment options for NL.

- **Global Skin:** An international alliance of dermatology patient organizations, advocating for patients' rights and promoting awareness.

- **Online Support Groups:** Platforms such as Reddit, Facebook, and dedicated forums where patients with NL can share experiences and advice.

- **ClinicalTrials.gov:** A database of ongoing clinical trials, offering information on the latest research studies related to NL.

- **Patient Advocacy Foundations:** Organizations like the Skin of Steel and The

Dermatology Foundation provide support and advocate for research funding.

Through continued education, advocacy, and support, we can enhance the lives of those living with Necrobiosis Lipoidica and move towards a future with better treatment options and ultimately, a cure.

www.ingramcontent.com/pod-product-compliance
Lightning Source LLC
Chambersburg PA
CBHW050646250726
48662CB00002B/520